This Book belongs to
Noralene Bebobose

WILD ANIMALS

A Collection of Photographs and Facts from the Animal Kingdom

An Interactive Book for Memory-Impaired Adults

Shadowbox Press books are designed to facilitate a rewarding reading experience by providing entertainment, education, and comfort to individuals diagnosed with Alzheimer's disease, Parkinson's disease, stroke, brain injury, or other memory-impairment condition.

For more information, go to www.shadowboxpress.com

Shadowbox Press, established in 2009, is an independent publisher committed to providing high-quality, interactive books to the memory-impaired adult audience.

Published by Shadowbox Press, LLC
P.O. Box 268
Richfield, OH 44286
www.shadowboxpress.com

Chief Creative Director: Matthew Schneider
Product Development Director: Deborah Drapac, BSN, RN

This book is intended to be informational and should not be considered a substitute for advice from a health care professional. The authors and the publisher expressly disclaim responsibility for any adverse effects arising from the use or application of the information contained in this book.

Publisher's Cataloging-in-Publication data

Schneider, Matthew John.
    Wild animals : a collection of photographs and facts from the animal kingdom, an interactive book for memory-impaired adults / Matthew Schneider ; Deborah Drapac, BSN, RN.
        p. cm.
        ISBN-13: 978-0-9831577-7-9; ISBN-10: 0-9831577-7-4
    1. Alzheimer's disease—Patients—Rehabilitation. 2. Dementia—Patients—Rehabilitation.
    3. Caregivers. 4. Self-care, Health. I. Drapac, Deborah Ann. I. Title.

RC523.S37 2011
362.196'831—dc22   2010917064

Manufactured in China

WILD ANIMALS

A Collection of Photographs and Facts from the Animal Kingdom

An Interactive Book for Memory-Impaired Adults

Matthew Schneider
Deborah Drapac, BSN, RN

3 1336 10901 0315

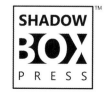

Shadowbox Press, LLC
Richfield, Ohio

INTRODUCTION

Shadowbox Press began with one simple mission: to develop interactive products for memory-impaired adults to revisit and share memories through the reading experience.

Storytelling is a valuable form of communication that connects one another and allows us to relate to each other on a personal level. It sparks the imagination, promotes self-reflection, and provides a way to find meaning in our experiences.

We have published a collection of books that offer a variety of subject matter designed to engage the user with meaningful content and provide a connection to both the past and present. Every effort has been made in the development of these books to maximize the experience for the user. They may be read independently or shared with an individual by a caregiver, loved one, staff member, or volunteer.

Our books offer a rewarding reading experience that stimulates the mind and offers engagement opportunities for the user. You will find inspiring words, inviting photographs, innovative conversation prompts, and unique activities to facilitate an interactive, multi-sensory experience. These books can generate meaningful communication and provide the feeling of well-being associated with sharing experiences and stories together. Through engagement, you may discover common backgrounds and interests, realize mutual bonds, and/or participate in a quality conversation.

We believe the reading experience should be shared at all stages of life, and sincerely hope that our passion for books touches your heart. We trust that you will find meaning, delight, and comfort in sharing a title from our collection of Shadowbox Press books. May you explore and discover memories, share experiences, and reflect on the value and purpose of life.

At Shadowbox Press, we welcome feedback from our readers and listeners. Please contact us at www.shadowboxpress.com to share your reading experiences, stories, and suggestions for future books.

ABOUT THIS BOOK

This book has been created to provide an interactive reading experience for a memory-impaired adult. It is designed to encourage socialization, evoke memories, prompt conversation, and supply mental and physical stimulation, thereby improving the overall quality of life for the individual user.

There are a variety of benefits from using this book. By encouraging engagement through personal reminiscing; a feeling of empowerment, an elevated mood, a positive self-image, and/or a reduced level of depression may result. In addition, a caregiver's presence, support, and attention can communicate acceptance, reassurance, and affection to a memory-impaired adult.

This book is comprised of three sections:

1. The STORY is the foundation of the book and is designed to entertain, inform, inspire, and/or educate. It features inviting photographs paired with engaging, large-print text written in clear, concise, and easy-to-read sentences. The content is intended to cultivate an interest in reading, evoke memories, and encourage opportunities to reminisce.

2. CONVERSATION STARTERS are questions that directly correlate to an individual set of pages from the STORY. Each series of inquiry-based questions are designed to prompt a dialog from experiences, events, and/or relationships. Engaging in conversation provides a memory-impaired adult the opportunity to share special memories and unique experiences from their life.

3. ACTIVITIES are exercises based on sensory stimulation, creative expression, and physical movement. These simple but purposeful activities correspond to the overall theme of the book, and are designed to provide additional mental and physical enrichment. Participation in a variety of activities is essential to overall good health and emotional well-being.

This book does not have to be read in its entirety to provide a benefit. Each set of pages is intended to encourage thinking, stimulate emotions, and evoke unique memories. An individual page may trigger a response and lead to a meaningful conversation. Through the reading and reminiscing process, the user can share his or her unique life story, express personal values, and, perhaps, reveal a legacy to pass on to future generations.

INTERACTION GUIDELINES

Communication is what connects us to each other. Because memory impairment slowly diminishes communication skills, it creates distinct challenges in how an individual communicates their thoughts and emotions, as well as comprehend what is being communicated to them. The key to managing the behaviors associated with memory impairment lies in the methods of engagement by caregivers and others. It is important to adapt our thinking and behaviors to create a more comfortable environment for a memory-impaired adult.

Guidelines for a successful reading experience:

- Locate a quiet, comfortable setting, free of distractions, for the reading experience.
- Before beginning, take a moment and allow yourself to relax. Imagine a connection between the voice and the story and reflect upon the importance of the time spent together.
- Always approach the individual from the front and make eye contact.
- Position your head at the same level as the individual's head. Bend your knees or sit down to reach a correct level.
- Smile whenever it's appropriate. A connection can grow from a smile.
- Present the book to the individual and invite them to share in the reading experience.
- Read aloud slowly, in an adult tone with a clear, calm, inviting, and enthusiastic voice, pausing after each sentence.
- Speak in short, direct sentences, focusing on a single idea at a time.
- Focus on central words and ideas, emphasizing the ones that may evoke memories.
- Point out key aspects of the photographs and invite the individual to share their thoughts.
- Include your own comments and encourage the individual to share their memories by prompting them with the CONVERSATION STARTERS.
- Ask only one question at a time, allowing the individual to answer it before continuing.
- Be aware of nonverbal cues. It is often possible to recognize a connection by observing facial expressions and/or body language.
- After a response, either verbal or nonverbal, acknowledge the contribution with positive reinforcement and encourage further discussion.
- Remember to be patient, as it may take longer for a memory-impaired adult to fully process and respond to a particular word, phrase, idea, or image.
- At times, engagement may become challenging. However, always treat the individual with dignity and respect.

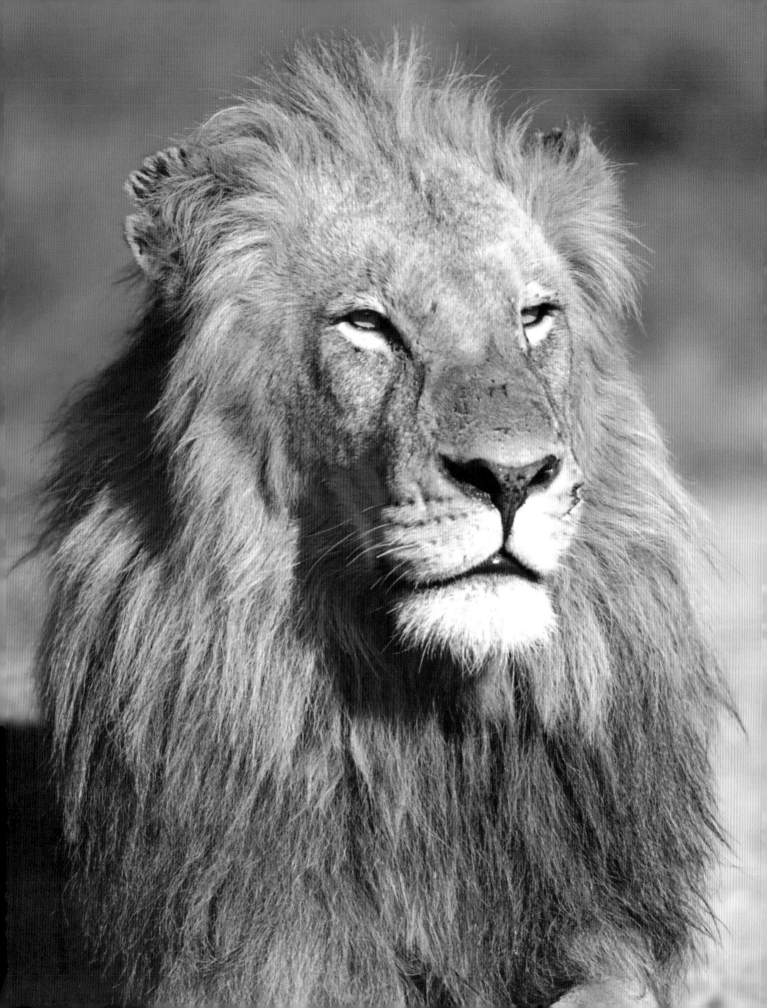

Lions are social animals within their communities. They are the only cats that live in groups called prides. In a pride, lions work together to hunt prey, raise cubs, and defend their territory.

Did you know?

The roar of a lion can be heard up to five miles away.

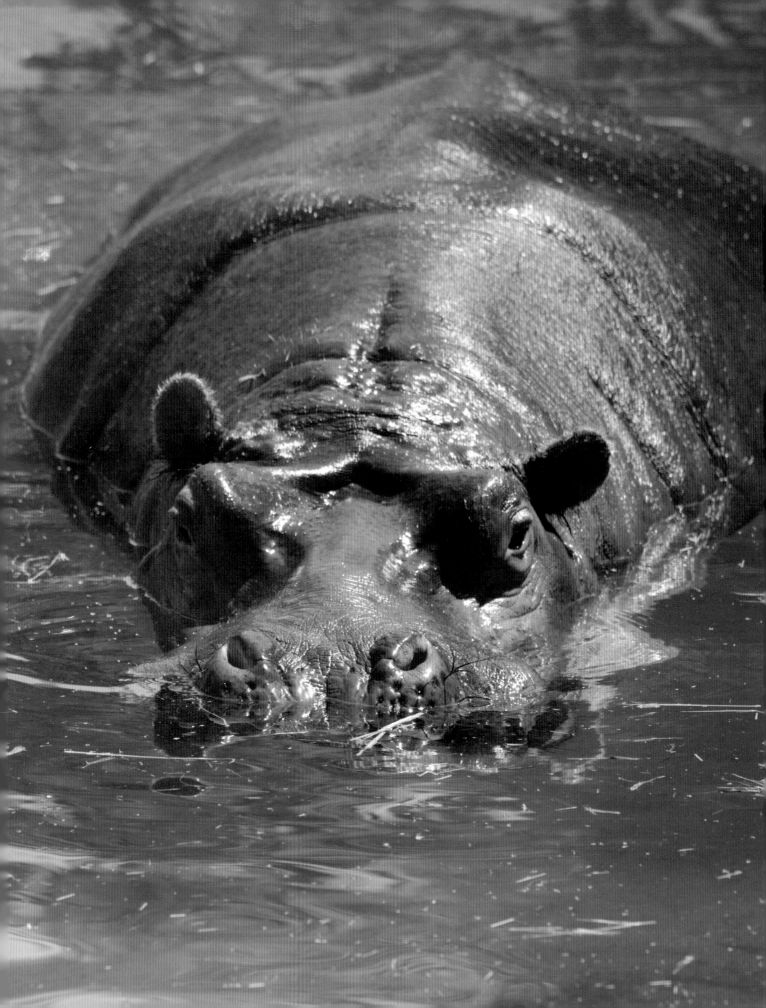

A **hippopotamus** is a large, plant-eating African mammal. Their eyes, ears, and nostrils are located high on the top of their heads. This allows hippos to remain submerged in water to stay cool and prevent sunburn in their tropical climate.

Did you know?

A hippopotamus can stay under water for up to 30 minutes.

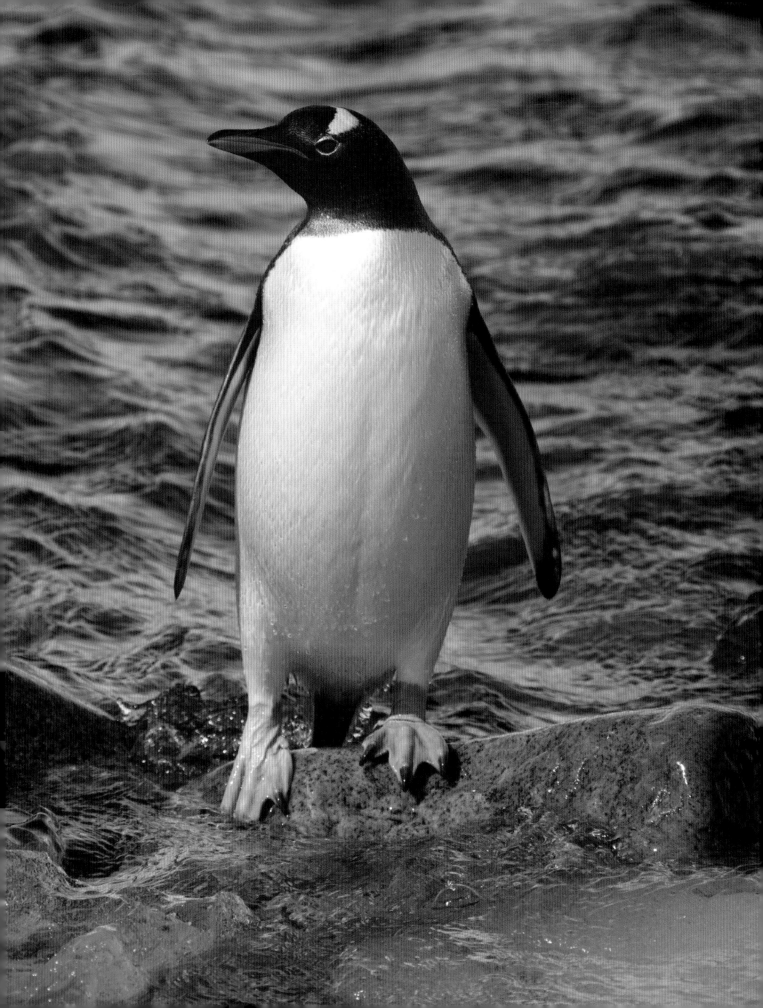

Penguins are flightless birds found in arctic climates. They have a thick, waterproof coat of feathers that insulates their entire body. In severe cold weather, penguins huddle together for warmth and protection.

Did you know?

A penguin can jump up to six feet high.

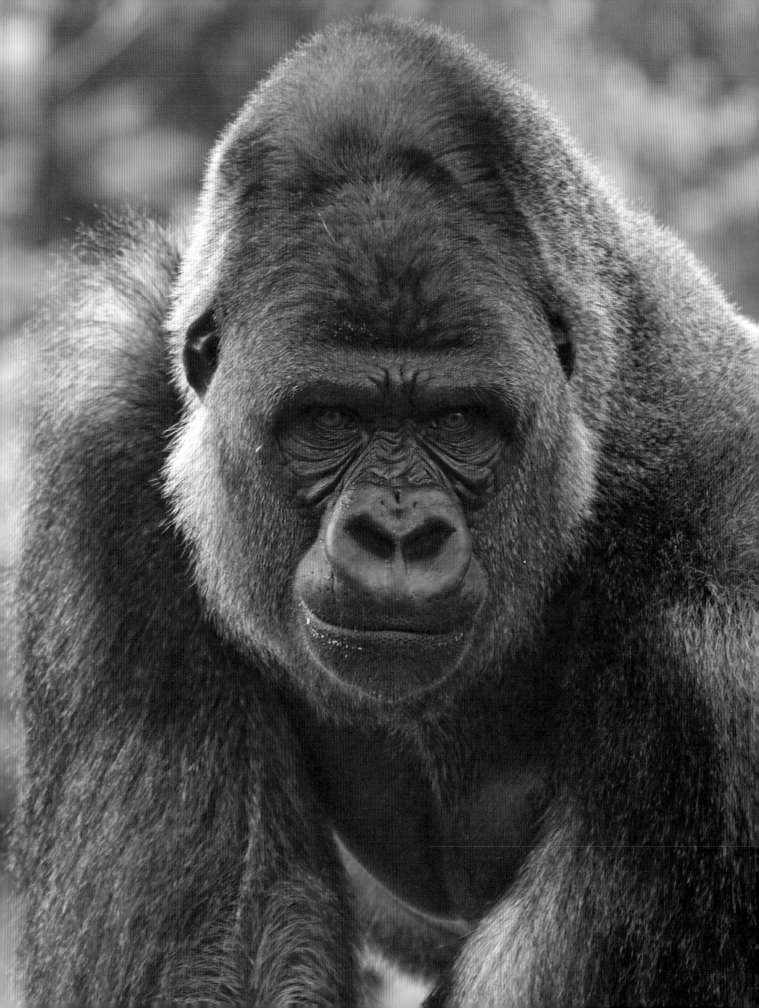

Gorillas are found in west central and east central Africa. They are peaceful, gentle, social, and mainly vegetarian mammals. Their occasional ferocious displays are generally from males protecting their families from threats.

Did you know?

An adult gorilla will eat more than 40 pounds of vegetation per day.

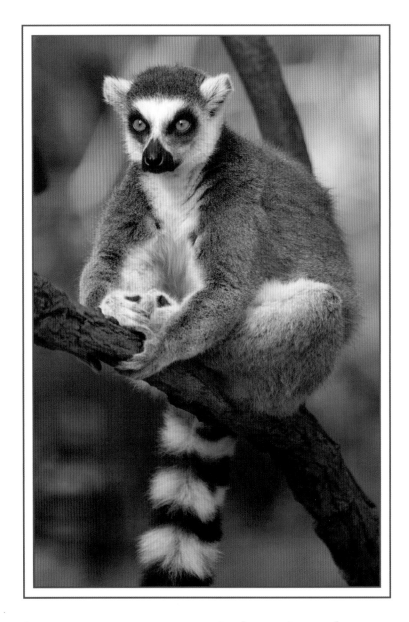

Lemurs are social animals with long limbs and noses, and flexible toes and fingers.

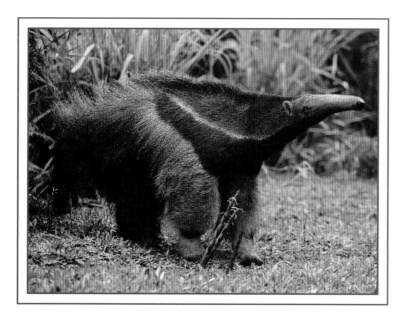

An **anteater** has no teeth, but its tongue can extend more than two feet to capture its prey.

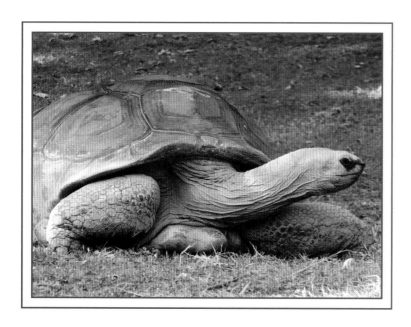

The oldest **tortoise** on record lived to be 152 years old.

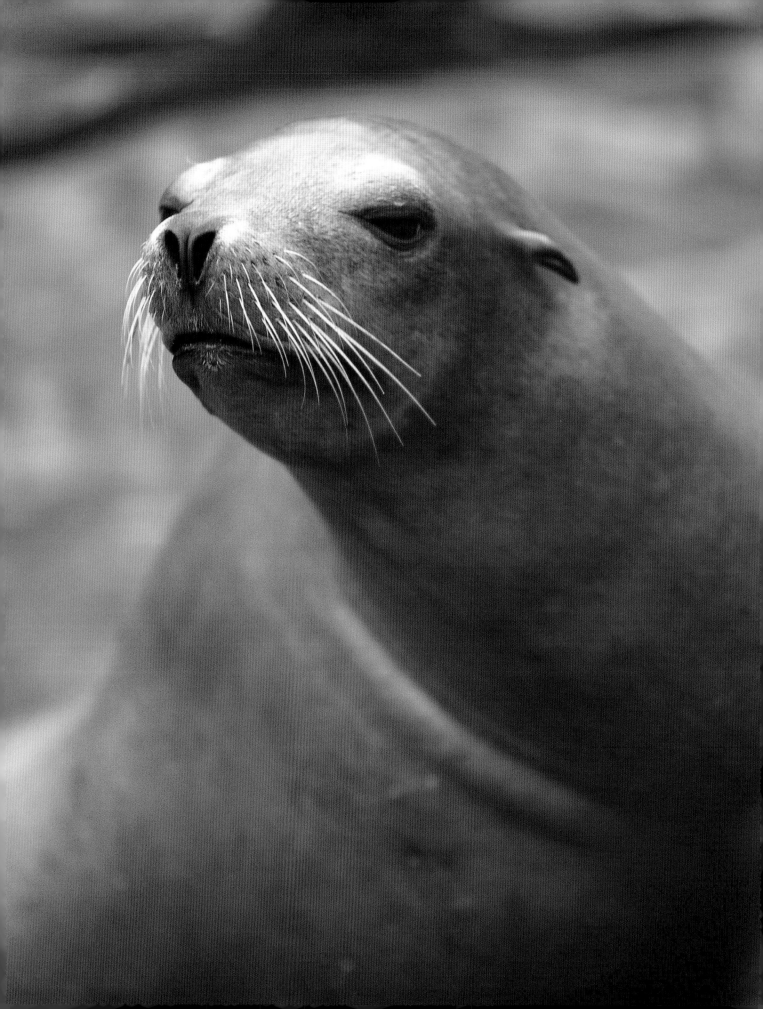

Seals have excellent eyesight and sensitive whiskers, which can detect the movement of nearby fish. Their sleek bodies move swiftly through the water, and their strong jaws and sharp teeth easily subdue fish, squid, and crustaceans.

Did you know?

A female seal is called a cow, and a male seal is called a bull.

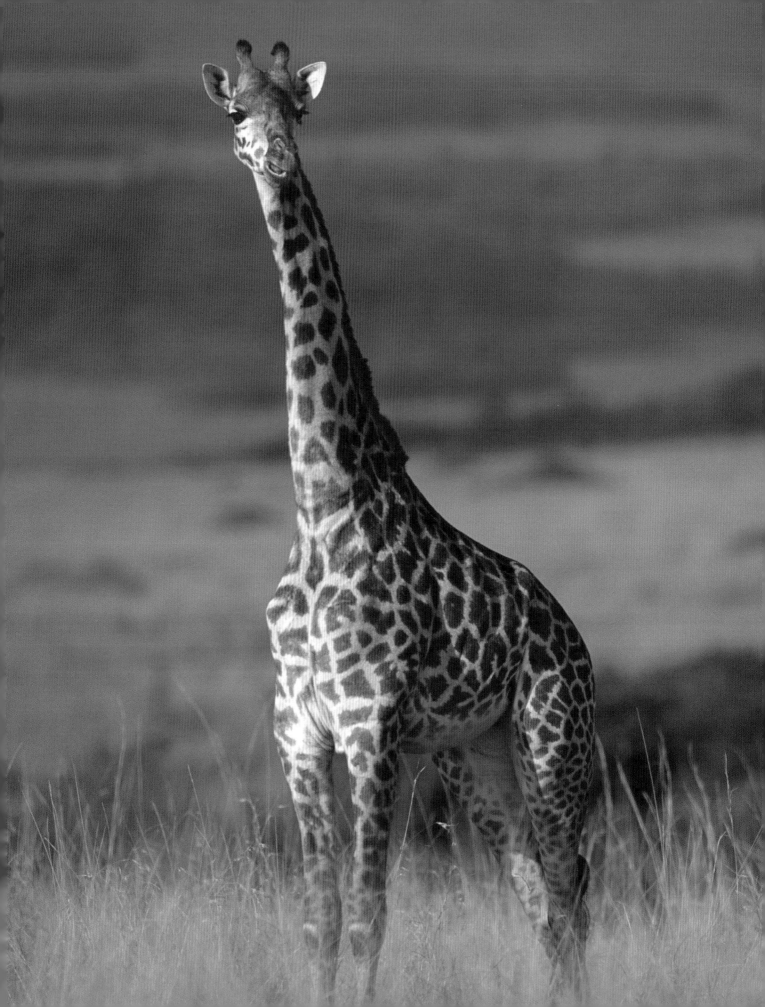

Giraffes are the tallest land mammals in the world. A male can grow up to 18 feet tall. Their height enables them to reach high into the acacia trees to feed. It also lets them see predators from great distances on the open grasslands.

Did you know?

A giraffe will sleep standing up and for only ten minutes to two hours per day.

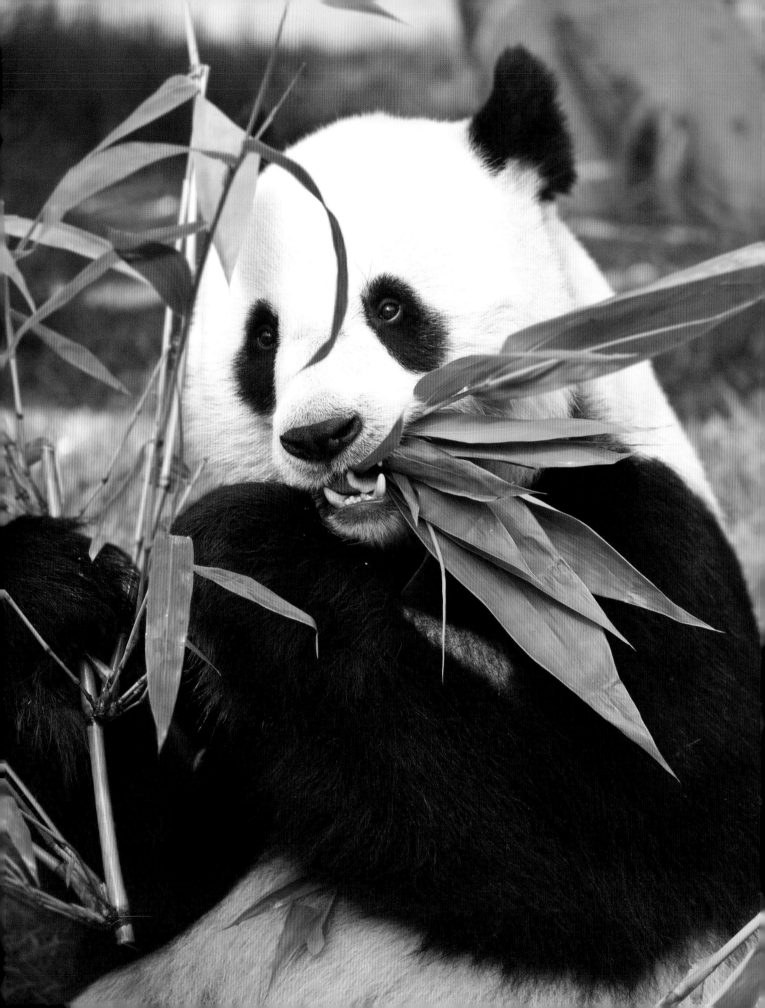

Pandas live in the remote, mountainous regions of central China. They are shy animals and spend most of their lives alone. Pandas feed on the shoots and leaves of bamboo plants. This accounts for 99 percent of their diet.

Did you know?

A typical panda spends 12 out of every 24 hours eating.

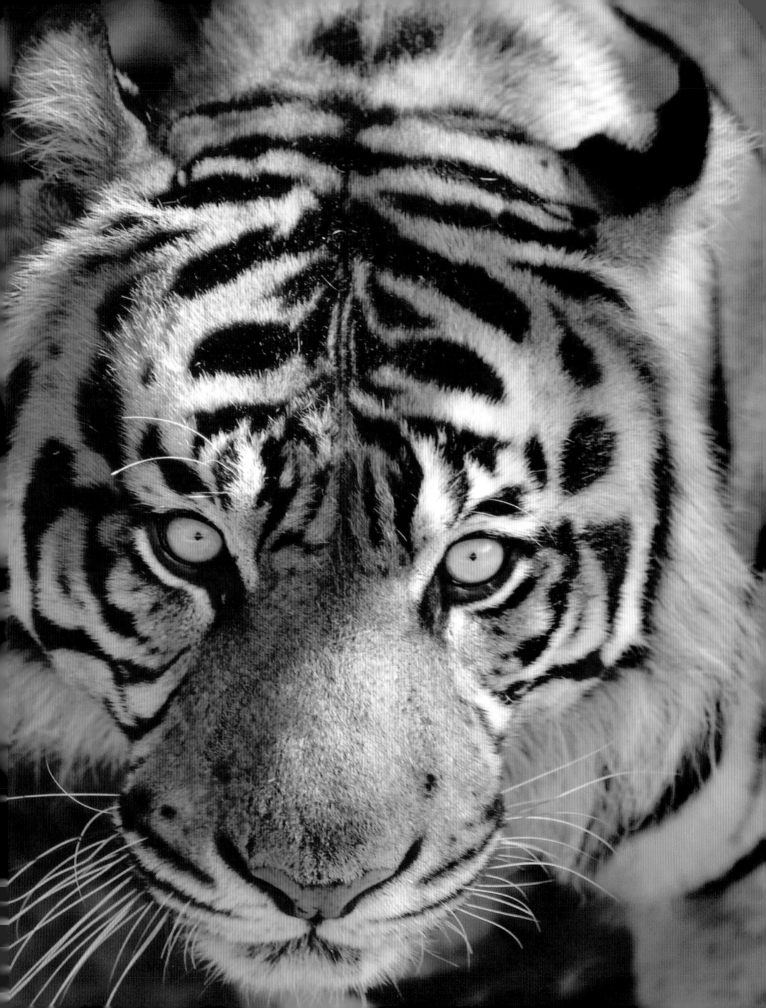

Tigers are the largest members of the cat family. They can weigh over 700 pounds and stretch up to six feet in length. These powerful predators usually hunt alone and are able to bring down prey such as buffalo, deer, and antelope.

Did you know?

A tiger has striped skin under its striped fur.

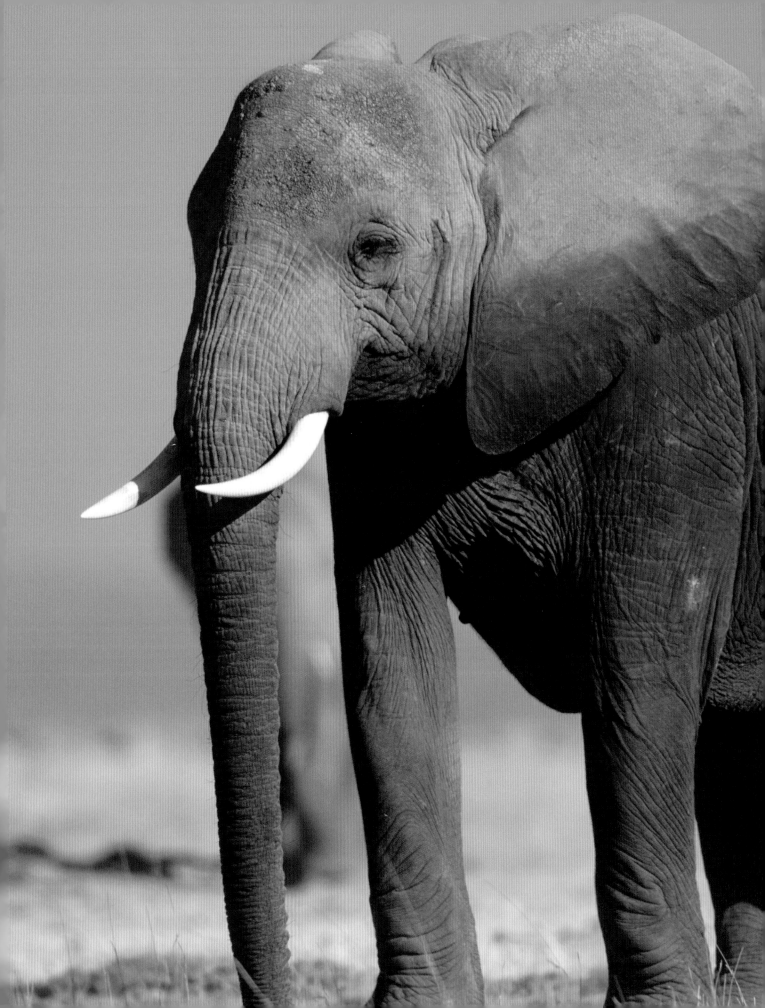

Elephants are the largest land mammals on Earth, weighing as much as 14,000 pounds. They are a symbol of wisdom in the Asian culture and are widely known for their great memory and intelligence.

Did you know?

An elephant can smell water up to three miles away.

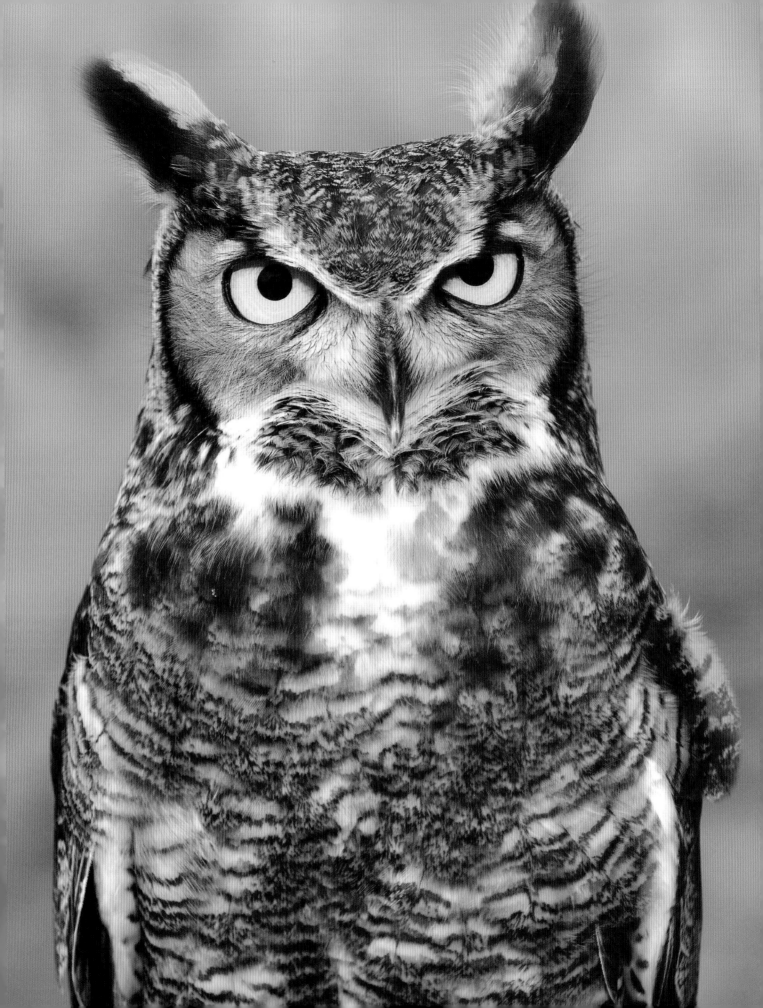

Owls are nocturnal, carnivorous birds.
They have powerful feet with sharp claws
for catching and holding their prey.
Owls feed on a variety of creatures,
including insects, birds, and small mammals.

Did you know?

An owl can turn its head 135 degrees
in either direction.

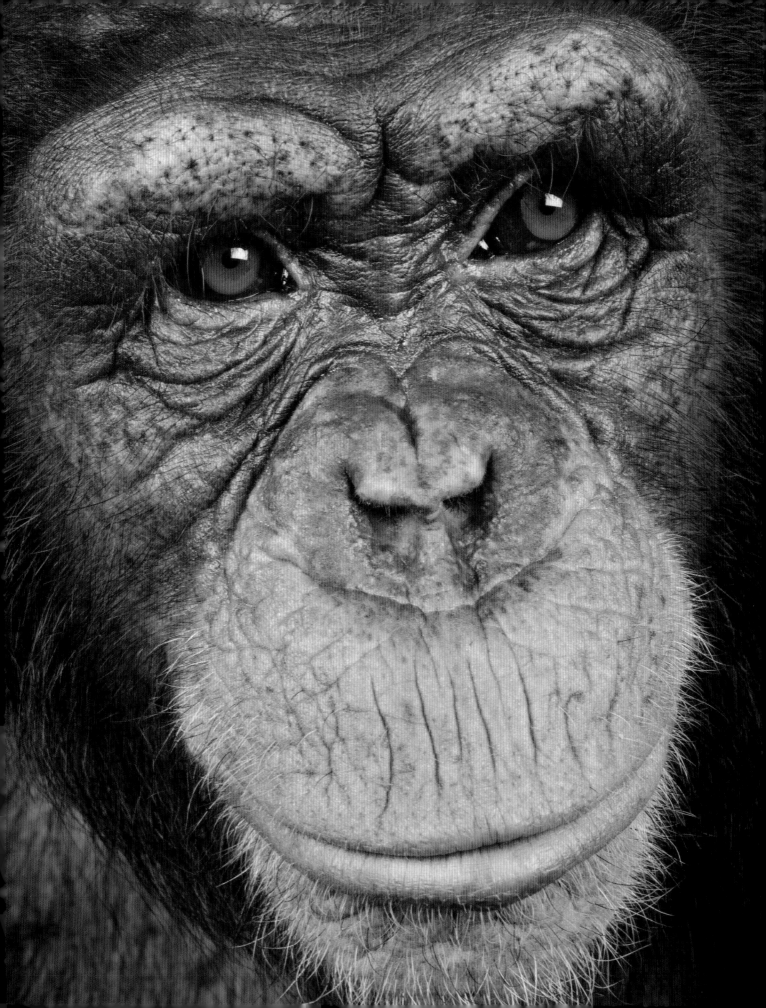

Chimpanzees live primarily in Africa. They are one of the few animals that use tools. Chimpanzees shape sticks to retrieve insects from their nests, use stones as hammers to open nuts, and use dried leaves as sponges to collect water for drinking.

Did you know?

A chimpanzee is the closest living relative to man.

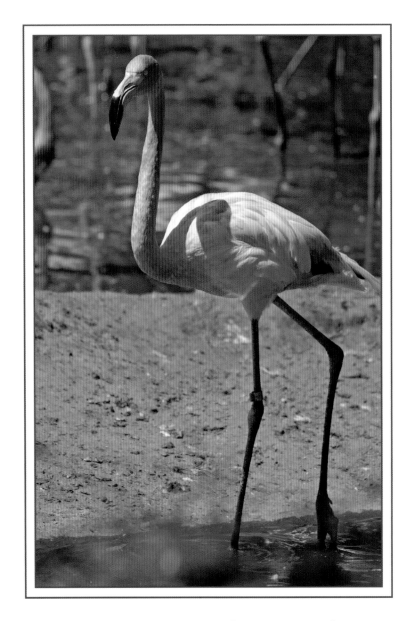

Flamingos get their pink color from the shrimp-like crustaceans they eat.

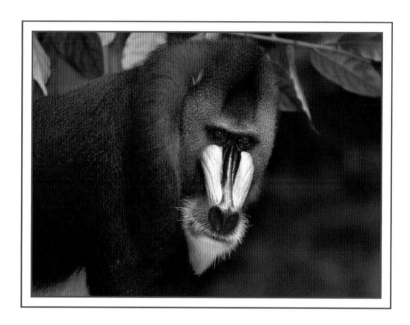

A **mandrill** is recognized by its bright blue rump, red-striped face, and yellow beard.

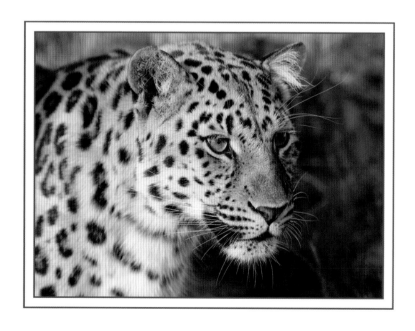

A **leopard's** dark spots are called rosettes, because they resemble the shape of a rose.

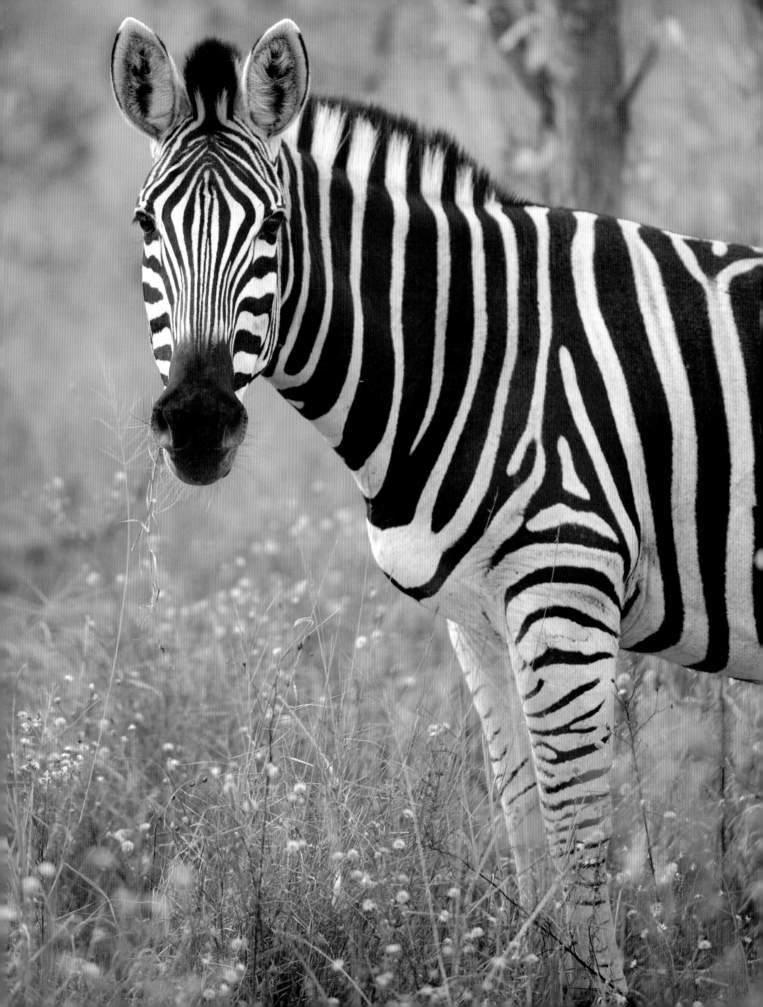

Zebras have a more distinctive coat than perhaps any other animal. Their stripes are as unique as fingerprints, with no two zebras having the exact same pattern. A zebra's stripes blend into vertical grasses, and many believe that they act as camouflage.

Did you know?

A baby zebra can stand within 20 minutes of being born and run when it is only an hour old.

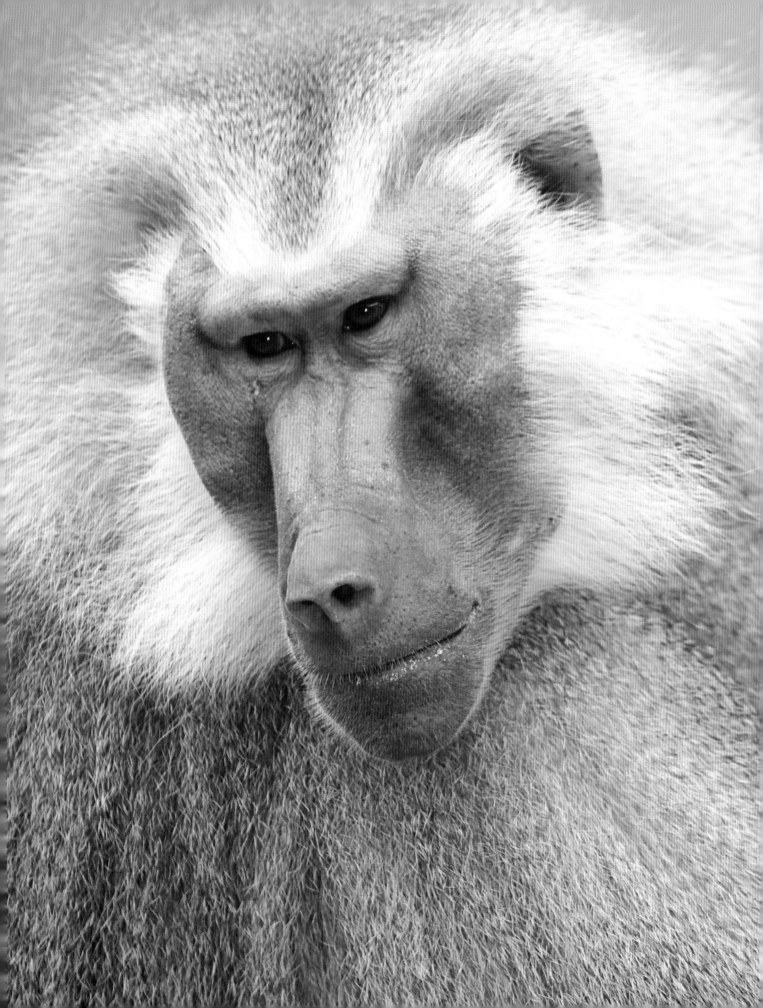

All **baboons** live in Africa or Arabia and are some of the world's largest monkeys. Friendship is very important in the baboon society. Their friendships may include sharing food, defense, and grooming one another to remove insects.

Did you know?

There are five different species of baboons.

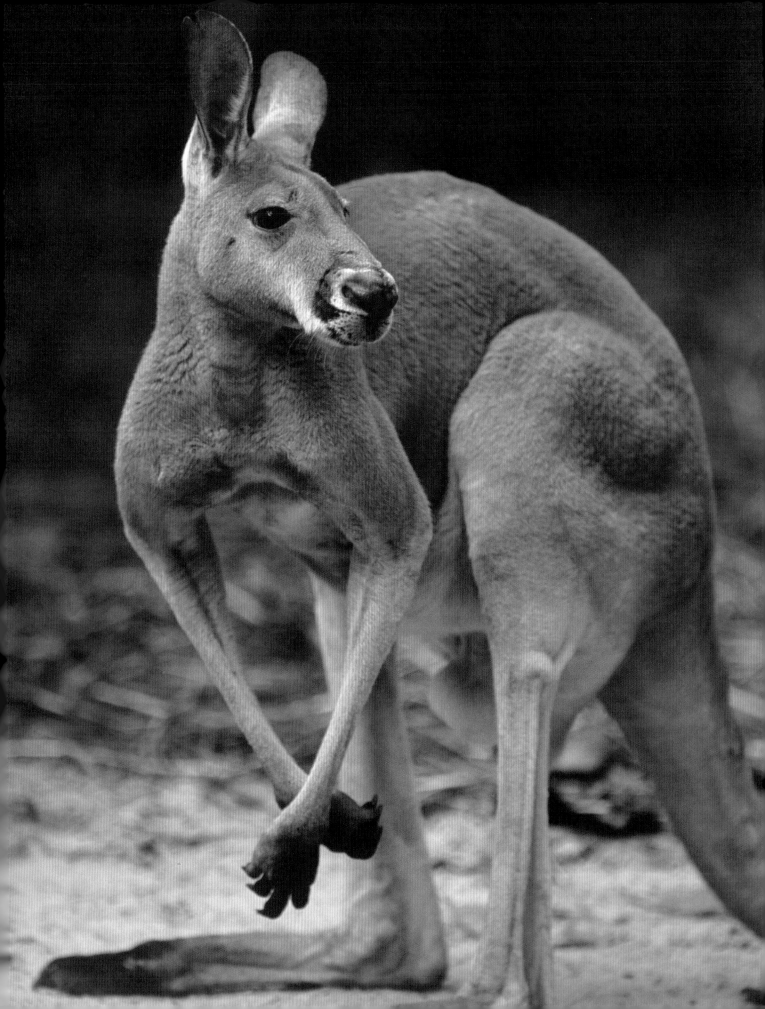

Kangaroos are marsupials. A marsupial is an animal that carries its young in a pouch. Kangaroos are the only animals that move by hopping. They hop on their powerful hind legs and use their tails for balance and steering.

Did you know?

A kangaroo cannot move backwards.

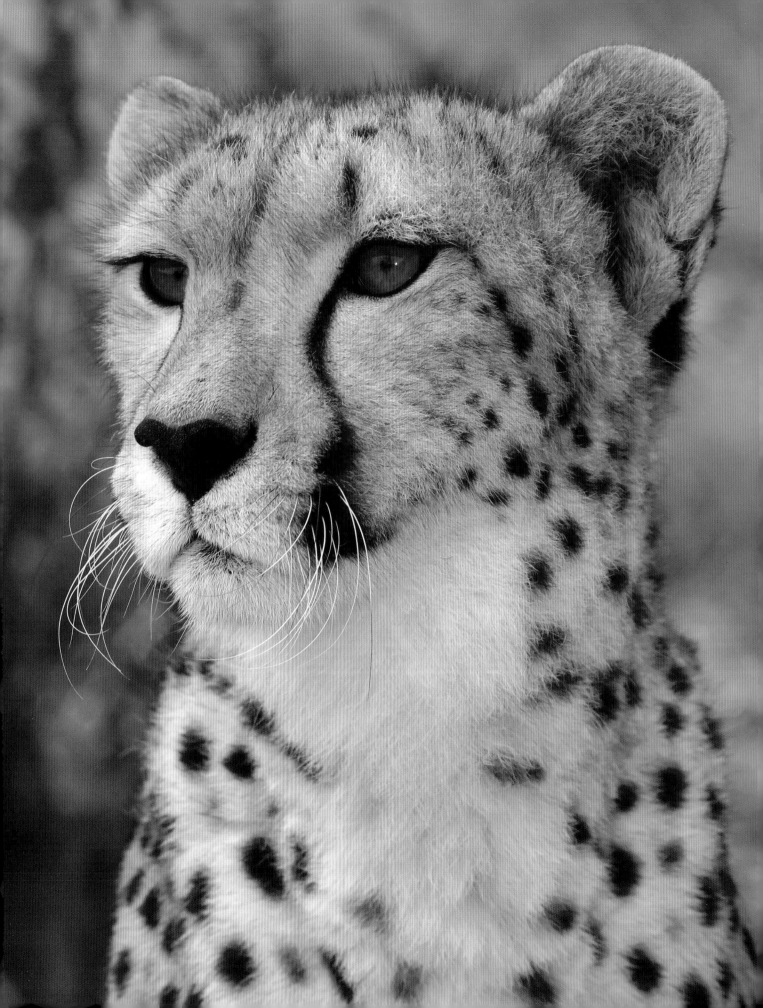

Most **cheetahs** are found in eastern and southwestern Africa. They are the fastest of all land animals and can reach speeds of more than 65 miles per hour. Cheetahs often perch in high places, where they, with their excellent eyesight, watch for prey.

Did you know?

The cheetah has been trained by man for hunting as far back as 3000 BC.

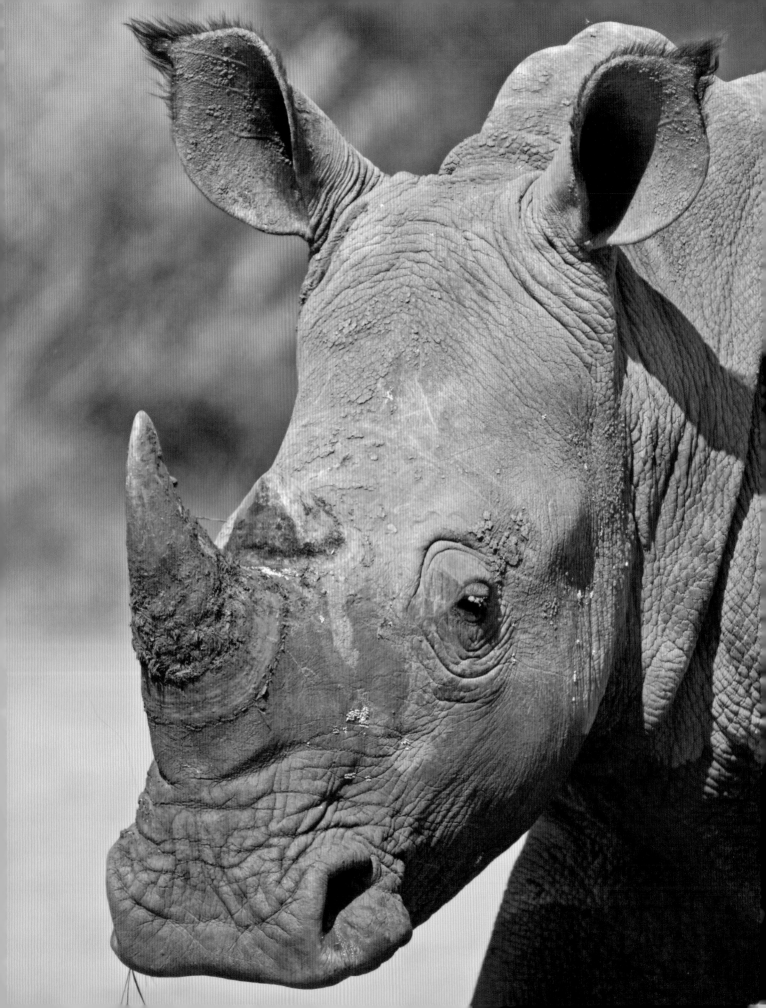

A **rhinoceros** has a keen sense of hearing and smell. However, they have poor eyesight and sometimes charge objects like trees or rocks, mistaking them as threats. A rhinoceros has no real threat. No other animal is a match for an adult rhino's heavily armored body of very thick skin and lethal horns.

Did you know?

A rhinoceros can live to be 50 or more years old.

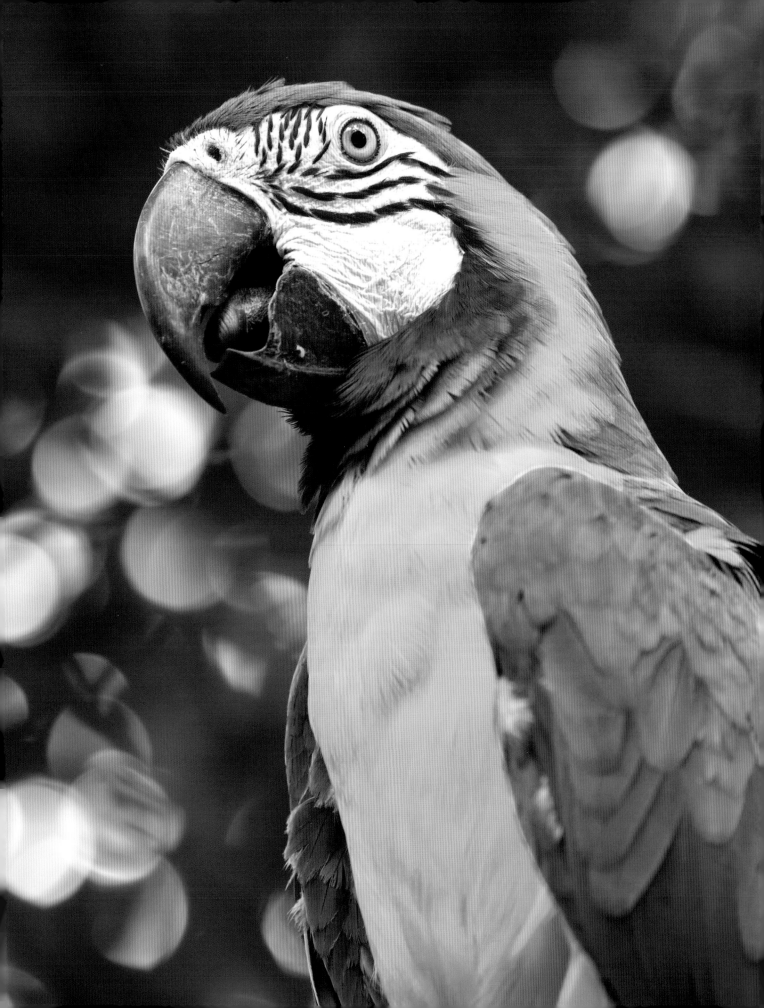

Parrots are found in warm climates over most of the world. The greatest numbers exist in Australia, Central America, and South America. They eat fruit, flowers, buds, nuts, seeds, and sometimes insects. Some parrots can mimic sounds, including human speech.

Did you know?

The average lifespan of a parrot in the wild is 80 years.

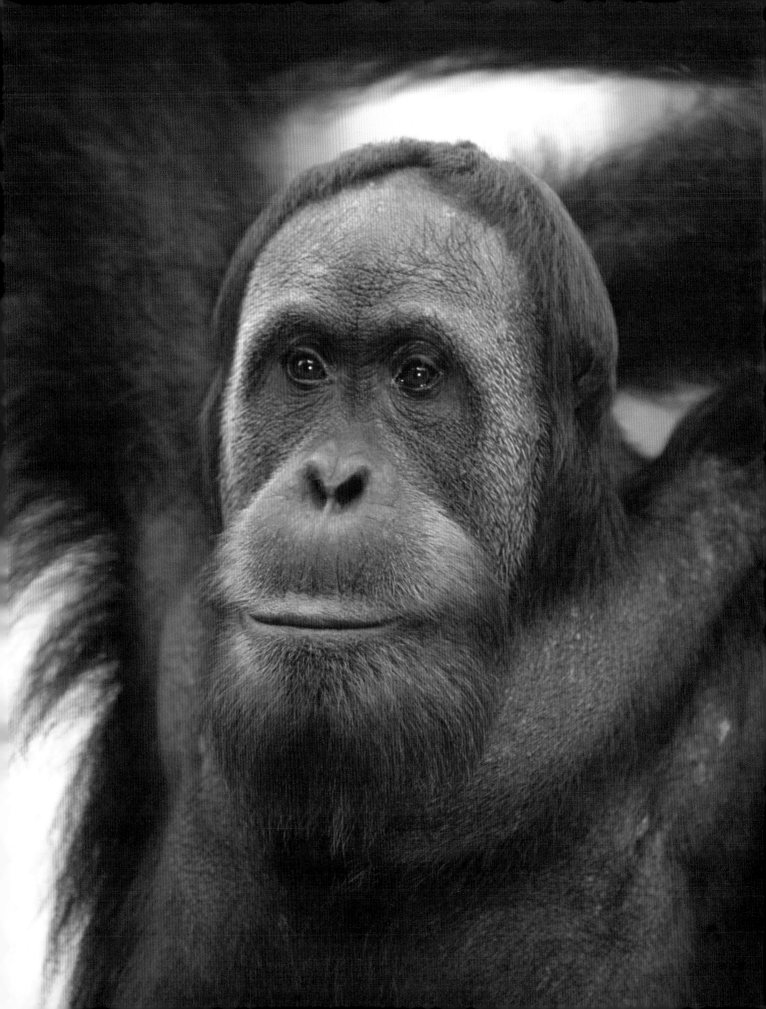

Orangutans are only found in the rainforests on the islands of Borneo and Sumatra. They are known for their intelligence, their reddish-brown hair, and long arms. An orangutan's powerful arms and hook-shaped hands and feet allow them to climb and swing from trees with ease.

Did you know?

The orangutan is the only great ape found outside of Africa.

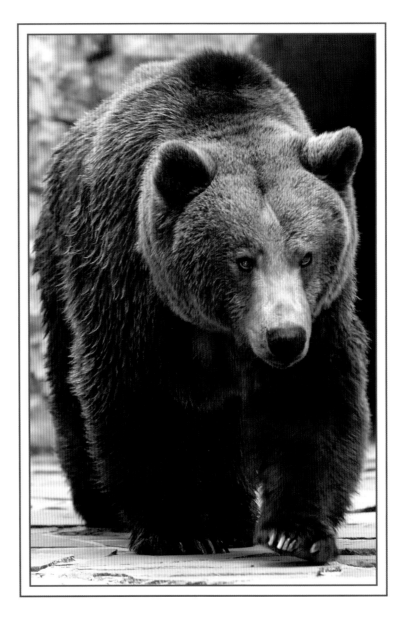

A **grizzly bear** is typically brown, though its fur can appear to be white-tipped or grizzled.

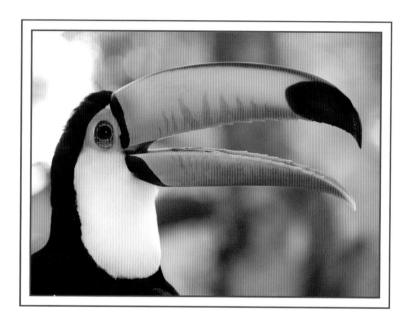

The **toucan's** oversized bill is better adapted for feeding than fighting.

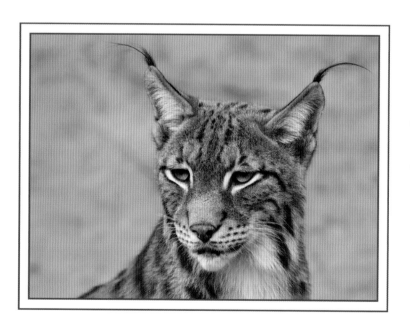

A **lynx** can spot a small animal up to 250 feet away.

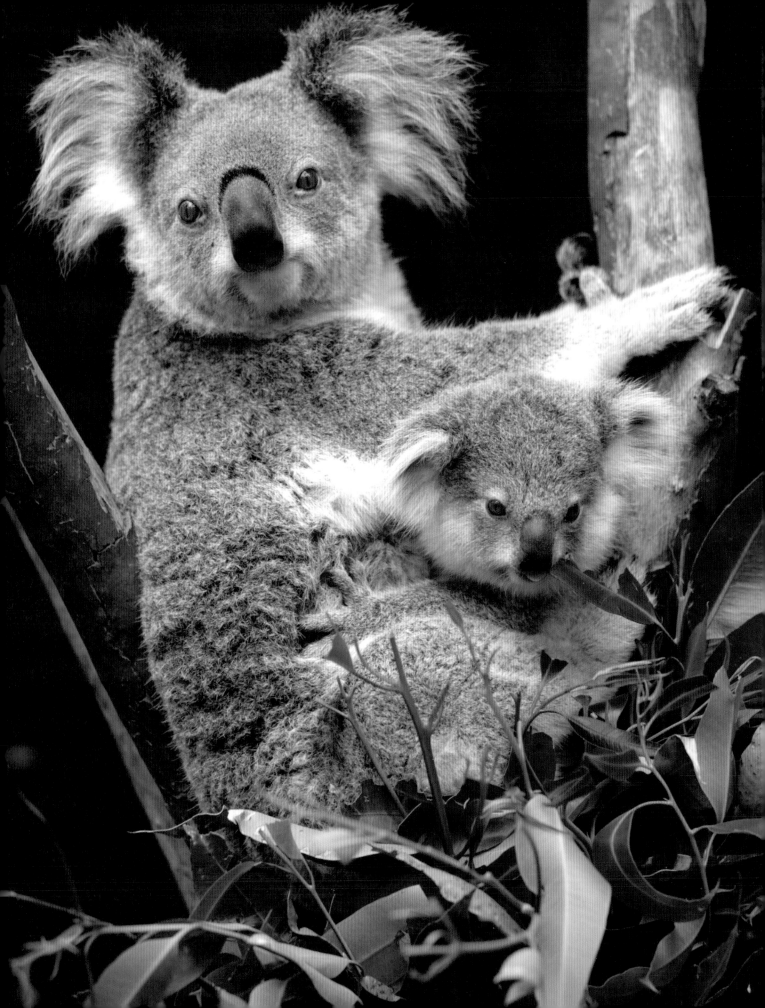

Koalas are often called "koala bears," but they are not bears at all. Like kangaroos, they are marsupials, or pouched mammals. Koalas live in eastern Australia, where the eucalyptus trees they feed on are most abundant.

Did you know?

The word "koala" means "no drink" because of the koala's ability to go many days without water.

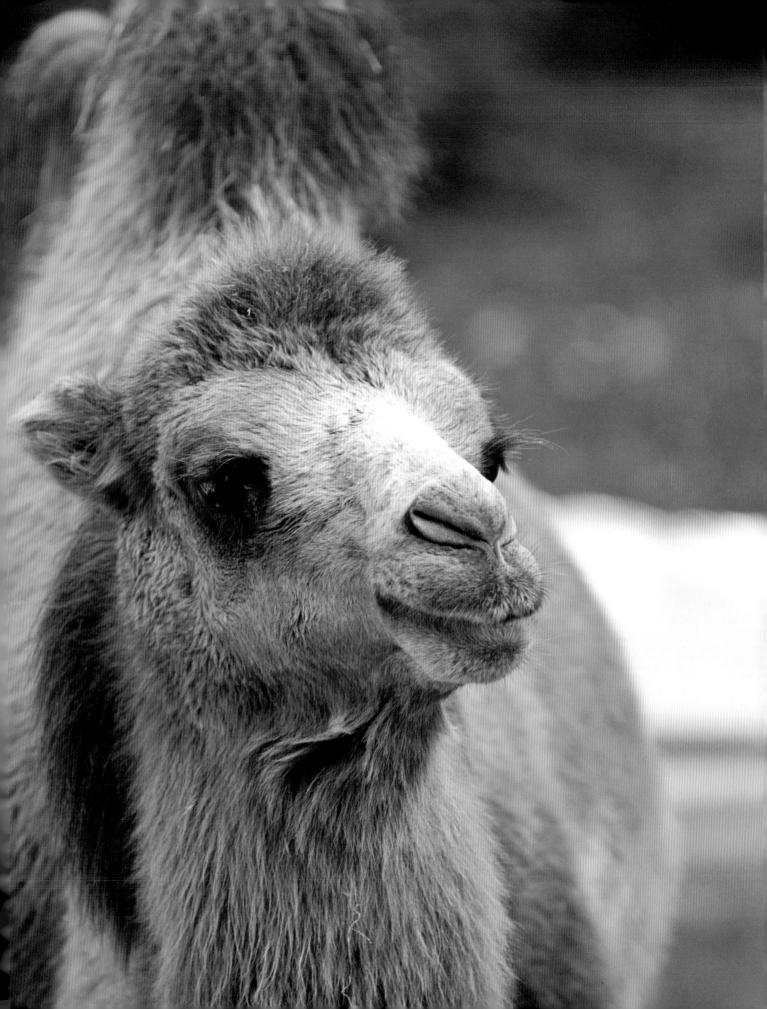

Camels can go for several days and travel up to 100 miles without food or water. A camel's hump can store as much as 80 pounds of fat, which is broken down into water and provides energy when nourishment is not available.

Did you know?

A camel has three eyelids to protect its eyes from the blowing sand.

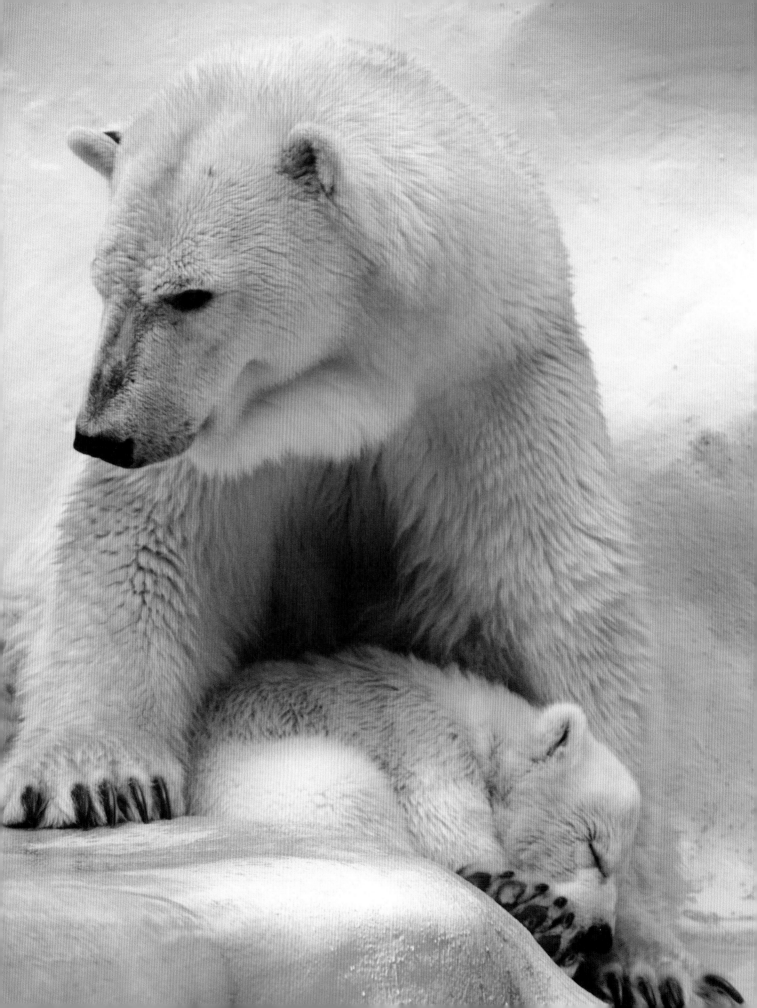

Polar bears live in the planet's coldest environments. Their thick coat of fur, which covers a layer of fat, insulates them against the cold. A polar bear's stark white or cream-colored coat provides camouflage from its prey in the surrounding ice and snow.

Did you know?

A polar bear can smell a seal up to two miles away?

CONVERSATION STARTERS
and ACTIVITIES

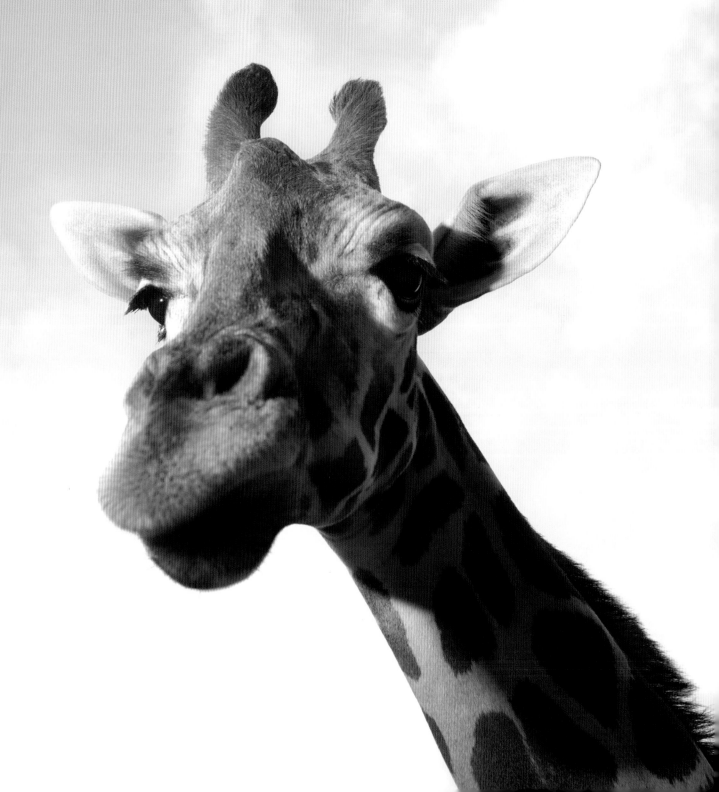

CONVERSATION STARTERS are designed to engage the user and encourage self-expression. They consist of a combination of close-ended (yes or no) and open-ended questions. Each series of questions correlate to an individual set of pages and are intended to be referenced during the reading experience. Each question is designed to prompt a response by the user from a photograph, word, phrase, or idea from the STORY. After a response from a specific question, either verbal or nonverbal, encourage further discussion on that particular subject. Urging the user to elaborate on an experience allows them to connect to the story and to the caregiver.

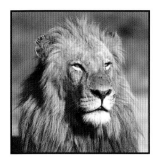

Did you know that a male lion is the only member of the cat family with a mane?

Have you ever seen a lion at the zoo?

Have you ever heard a lion roar?

What did you do as a child that required courage?

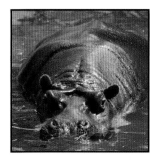

Did you know that a baby hippopotamus can weigh up to 100 pounds at birth?

Did you ever sunbathe in the summer?

Do you have any children or grandchildren?

What zoo animals did you like as a child?

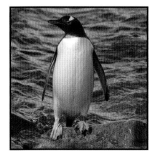

Did you know that a penguin can dive deeper underwater than any other bird?

Have you ever gone ice skating?

Did you walk to school in the winter when you were a child?

Where did you see animals when you were growing up?

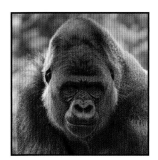

Did you know that a gorilla is six times stronger than a human?

Have you ever lifted weights?

Have you ever watched a movie featuring a gorilla?

What vegetables did you like to eat as a child?

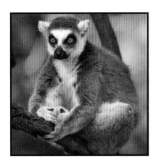

Did you know that lemurs live on the African island of Madagascar and some neighboring islands?

Did you know that an anteater uses its sense of smell to find anthills?

Did you know that a tortoise likes to spend the warmest part of the day underground?

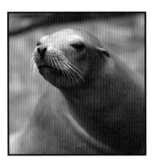

Did you know that a seal can hold its breath underwater for over 20 minutes?

Have you ever seen a seal balance a ball on its nose?

Did you ever dive into a swimming pool when you were growing up?

What beaches have you visited on vacation?

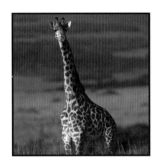

Did you know that the front legs of a giraffe are longer than its back legs?

Have you ever seen a giraffe eat leaves from a tree?

Is anyone in your family over six feet tall?

How did you reach for things when you were a small child?

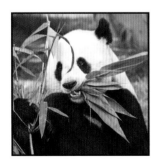

Did you know that the panda bear is popular in Chinese art?

Did you visit the bears at the zoo when you were a child?

Do you like to eat Chinese food?

What kind of stuffed animals did you have when you were a child?

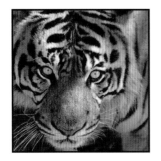

Did you know that a tiger is the only member of the cat family with striped fur?

Have you ever had a cat for a pet?

Did you like to read books about animals when you were growing up?

How many people are in your family?

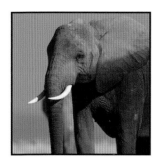

Did you know that an elephant is pregnant for 22 months before it gives birth?

Have you ever seen an elephant at the circus?

Have you ever fed an elephant peanuts at the zoo?

What animal shows did you watch on television when you were growing up?

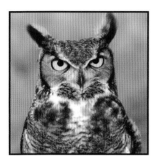

Did you know that an owl can see better at night than any other bird or animal?

Have you ever heard an owl in your neighborhood?

Did you like to stay up late at night when you were a child?

Who in your family liked to share their wisdom?

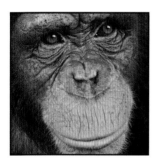

Did you know that a chimpanzee uses facial expressions to show love, surprise, and anger?

Have you ever seen a chimpanzee swinging from trees at the zoo?

Did you like to climb on monkey bars when you were a child?

What tools did your father use?

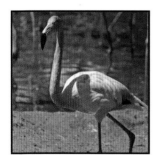

Did you know that a flamingo stands on both legs to eat and on one leg to rest?

Did you know that a male mandrill is the most colorful of all mammals?

Did you know that a leopard can climb a 50-foot-tall tree?

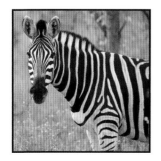

Did you know that a zebra sleeps standing up like a horse?

Have you ever driven a car through a wild animal park?

Have you ever worn a striped suit or striped dress?

What black-and-white movies do you like to watch?

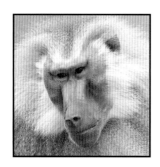

Did you know that a baboon can live in a group of up to 200 animals?

Did your parents ever have relatives or friends over for dinner?

Did you have fun playing with your friends when you were a child?

What hairstyles were popular when you were growing up?

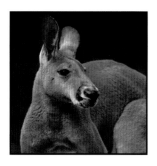

Did you know that a baby kangaroo is called a "joey"?

Did you ever walk backwards when you were a child?

Did you like to play hopscotch when you were growing up?

What kind of things do you keep in your pockets?

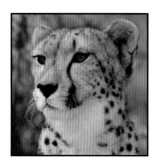

Did you know that a cheetah does not roar, but purrs like a domestic cat?

Could you run fast when you were a child?

Were you ever on the track team at school?

What playground games did you play when you were in school?

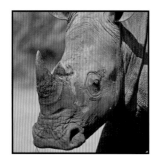

Did you know that the ears of a rhinoceros can turn in all directions?

Did you like learning about animals when you were in school?

Did you like to listen to the radio when you were a teenager?

What types of music do you enjoy?

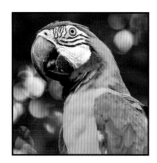

Did you know that a parrot can have green, red, yellow, or blue feathers?

Have you ever heard a parrot talk?

Have you ever had a bird for a pet?

What bright colors do you like?

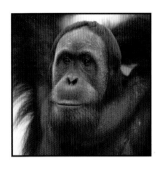

Did you know that an orangutan is sometimes called a "red ape"?

Did you have a swing in your yard when you were a child?

Have you ever been to an island?

Who do you know that has red hair?

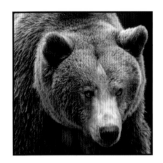

Did you know that a grizzly bear gains as much as three pounds a day as it prepares for hibernation?

Did you know that a toucan's bill can be four times larger than its head?

Did you know that a lynx has tufts of hair on the tips of its ears that enhance its hearing?

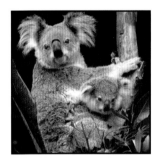

Did you know that a koala travels by leaping from tree to tree?

Did you like to climb trees when you were a child?

Have you ever had a eucalyptus cough drop?

What time did you go to bed when you were a child?

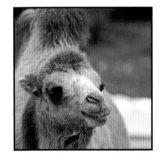

Did you know that a camel can drink 30 gallons of water in less than 15 minutes?

Have you ever seen anyone ride a camel?

Have you ever been to a very warm place?

What do you like to drink when you're thirsty?

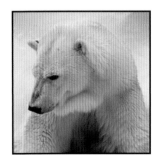

Did you know that a male polar bear can grow up to ten feet tall?

Do you like cold weather?

Have you ever gone ice fishing?

What special meals did your mother cook in the winter?

ACTIVITIES are designed to enrich the user's life by introducing diversity into the daily routine through mental and physical engagement. They are intended to be performed under the supervision of a caregiver. Caution should be exercised when outdoors, in unfamiliar surroundings, or when using potentially harmful materials and/or equipment. Selection of an appropriate activity is dependent on individual ability; however, the user may participate or benefit from observing another individual perform the activity.

SENSORY STIMULATION ACTIVITIES

Grow an elephant ear plant. Purchase a plant with 3–4 shoots and re-pot it in an 18-inch pot. Water and fertilize the plant and place it in an area that receives a lot of sunlight. Allow the plant to mature to 10–15 stalks and enjoy its large, richly-colored leaves.

Make a pine cone bird feeder. Coat a pine cone with a generous amount of peanut butter. Pour some birdseed in a shallow pan and roll the pine cone in the birdseed until it's completely covered. Attach a string to the pine cone feeder and hang it in a tree for the birds to enjoy.

Get a book of animal jokes or riddles. Reading and telling jokes is fun for people of all ages. Good, healthy laughter helps reduce stress, diminish pain, and increase energy. Enjoy laughing and bringing smiles to others.

Bake monkey bread. Monkey bread is a sticky, gooey pastry traditionally served at breakfast. Locate a quick and easy monkey bread recipe and prepare it as directed. Serve it warm so that it can be easily torn apart with the fingers and eaten by hand.

Listen to a nature sounds CD. Start the CD, close both eyes, and escape to a paradise filled with natural sounds of the environment. Relive memories of relaxing outdoors, enjoying wildlife, and taking fun-filled vacations.

Visit an art museum. Animals have been depicted in art for thousands of years. Identify artwork of animals from a variety of periods. Explore paintings, sculptures, and ceramics while discovering how animals have influenced art throughout history.

Look at a world map or globe. Maps are interesting and educational. Study the continents, countries, islands, and oceans. Locate and discuss animal habitats from around the world.

Purchase a stuffed animal. Select a realistic and cheerful animal. Stuffed animals are comforting to hold, squeeze, and cuddle. They can reduce stress and loneliness, and they are therapeutic for arthritic hands. Experience the companionship and security a stuffed animal can provide.

Have a movie matinee. Darken a room in the afternoon and watch a movie with an animal, jungle, or safari theme. Make hot-buttered popcorn and enjoy a cold drink to more closely imitate the movie-going experience.

CREATIVE EXPRESSION ACTIVITIES

Paint with a feather. Paint a picture on a large piece of drawing paper using all the parts of a feather. Use india ink and the quill end of the feather to create sharp lines. Use the feather tip and the feather web with poster paints to create soft, sweeping areas of color. When finished, discuss the emotions the painting evokes.

Make a dried eucalyptus flower arrangement. Secure a foam block inside a vase. Trim the eucalyptus branches to create varying heights and begin placing them into the foam block. Once the branches are in place, step back and look at the arrangement from all angles. If needed, fill in any sparse areas. Enjoy the beauty and fragrance of the arrangement.

Make an animal print. Choose an animal print to replicate. Cut a sponge in the shape of an animal's spot or stripe. Paint the entire paper the background color of the skin with tempera paint and allow it to dry. Dip the sponge in the paint and dab it onto the paper to create the desired pattern. Enjoy exploring the print-making process as an artistic medium.

Create an animal with clay. Choose an animal to make with a non-toxic modeling clay. For two-dimensional animals, flatten the clay using a rolling pin and cut out the basic shape with an animal cookie cutter. For three-dimensional animals, roll and form the parts using the clay.

Paint a birdhouse. Purchase a small, unfinished birdhouse from a craft store. Paint it with an acrylic paint and then top-coat it with two coats of a water-based clear varnish. Use the birdhouse as an accent piece in a room or mount it outdoors.

PHYSICAL MOVEMENT ACTIVITIES

Take a trip to the zoo. Call the local zoo and inquire about opportunities for seniors. Many zoos offer programs and/or guided tours designed especially for senior citizens. Observe the animals and their unique habitats. Bring binoculars to examine the animals and a camera to capture memories of the day.

Take a winter nature walk. Look in the freshly fallen snow for animal tracks and bird footprints. Try to identify the prints and take notes to record the observations. Explore the fascinating world of nature in the winter.

Start an ornamental grass garden. Select an area that gets six hours of sunlight per day. Plant grasses such as blue fescue, quaking grass, and switchgrass. Grasses do not need fertilizer, but they do need to be watered regularly. Trim the grasses periodically to maintain their health.

Visit a natural history museum. A natural history museum is a great place to explore the many facets of Earth. Get acquainted with the area's native wildlife, learn about space and distant planets, and experience the massive, awe-inspiring dinosaurs that once ruled the planet.